YUCK!

Do I have to
EAT THAT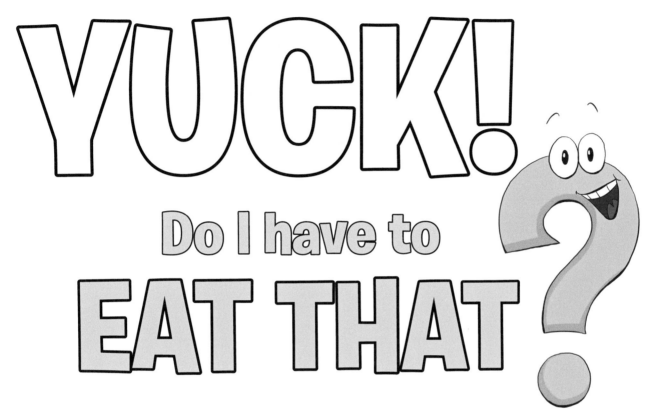

Are grown-ups just saying this or is it
really important that I eat healthily?

ALVINA FOO
PHARMACIST BPHARM (USYD)

Balboa Press books may be ordered through booksellers or by contacting:

Balboa Press
A Division of Hay House
1663 Liberty Drive
Bloomington, IN 47403
www.balboapress.com.au
1 (877) 407-4847

ISBN: 978-1-5043-1835-8 (sc)
ISBN: 978-1-5043-1836-5 (e)

Print information available on the last page.

Balboa Press rev. date: 07/17/2019

BALBOA
PRESS
A DIVISION OF HAY HOUSE

Acknowledgements

"A fun and interactive comic that will engage children and help them understand why it is important to eat healthy food."

DR. LEILA MASSON
Paediatrician & Lactation Consultant
Sydney, Australia

"I simply LOVE it!"

Dr Min Yeo
Medical Doctor
Sydney, Australia

"Alvina introduces your kids to good nutrition through simple and funny illustrations and points out the difference between nourishing whole foods and bad processed goods. This book is great for your young family and health educators."

Dr Suzi Wigge
Integrative Medicine GP
Sydney, Australia

"A fun and entertaining book to helping kids connect facts into good meal time choices. But it is also for the adult in understanding gut health. This is one of the greatest gifts you can give to anyone at any age!"

Dr Laurena Law
Integrative and Functional Medicine Doctor - Hong Kong

"LOL. The hilarious illustrations not only got my kids bursting out in laughters but also nodding their heads in agreement to the message of the book. Indeed laughter is always part of Good Medicine. Well done Alvina"

Dr Melanie Phuah
Lifestyle Medical Doctor, Singapore

"I love this book it's brilliant!

A fun insightful easy read encouraging health and wellness starting from within. Healthy gut, healthy mind, healthy body, soul and spirit!"

Chef Andre Sickinger
Beverly Hills LA

What Is Healthy Eating?

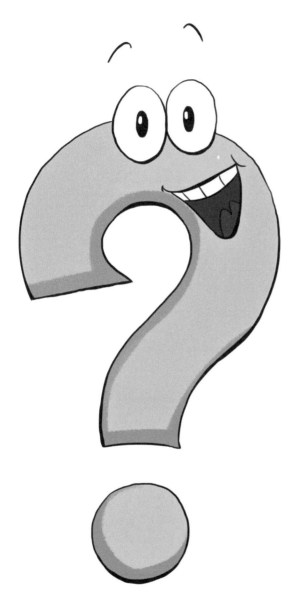

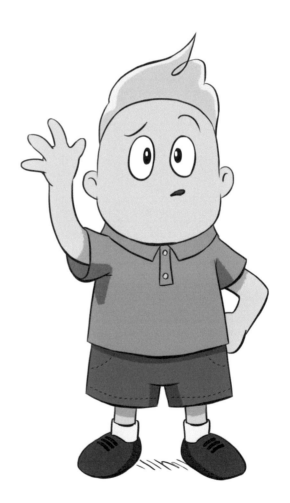

Fresh fruit

Lots of
different
veggies

Drinking
water

Ice-cream? Ahh...
I don't think so!

So... why is healthy eating important?

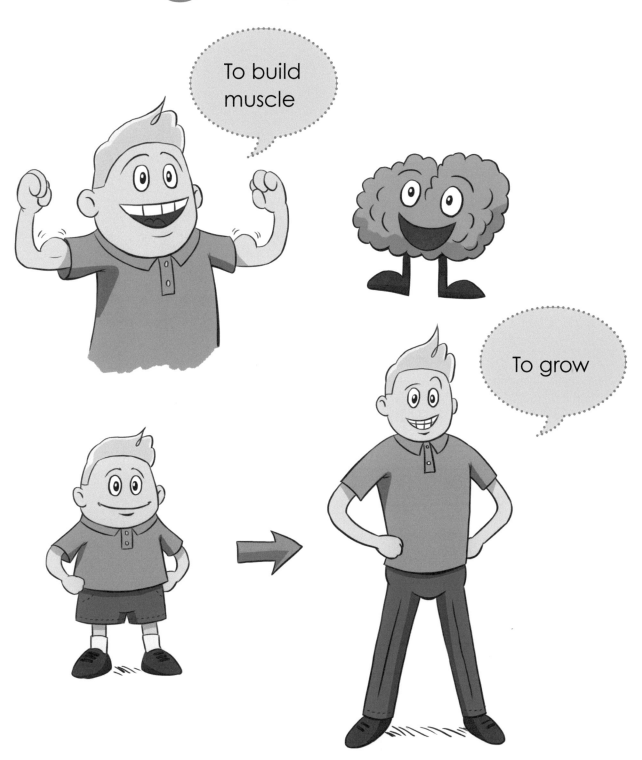

heart

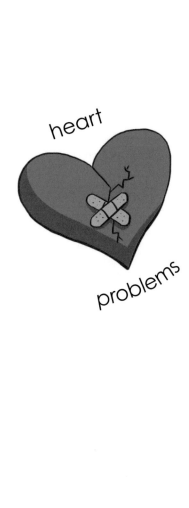

problems

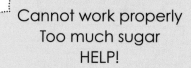

Cannot work properly
Too much sugar
HELP!

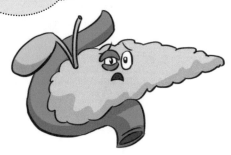

Pancreas

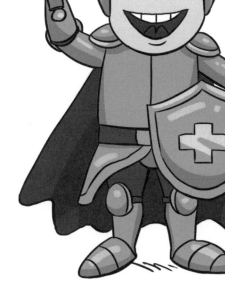

I like to
make you
feel sick!
Ha! Ha! Ha!

overweight

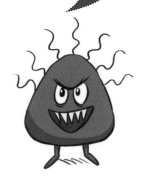

Infections

To Prevent Many Health Problems

But How?

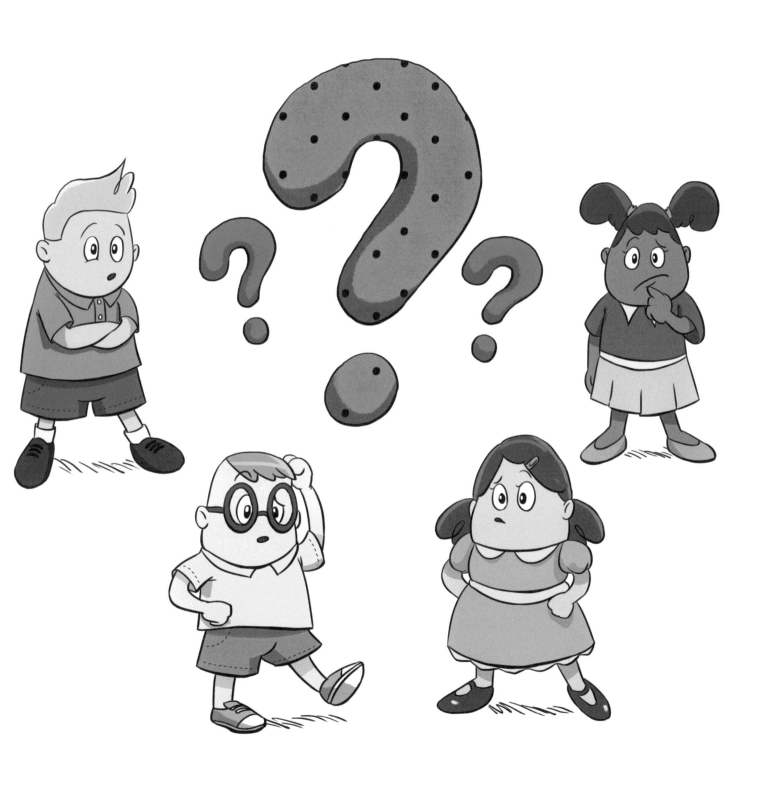

First... We need to look at the Human Body

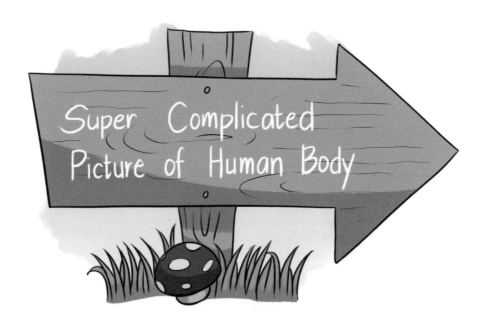

PRESENTING...
THE HUMAN BODY!!!

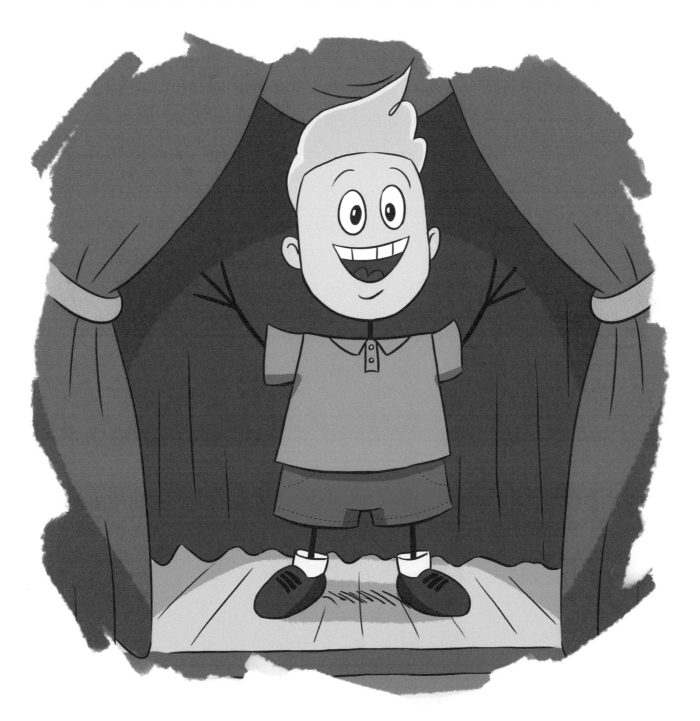

I told you that it's complicated!

Question

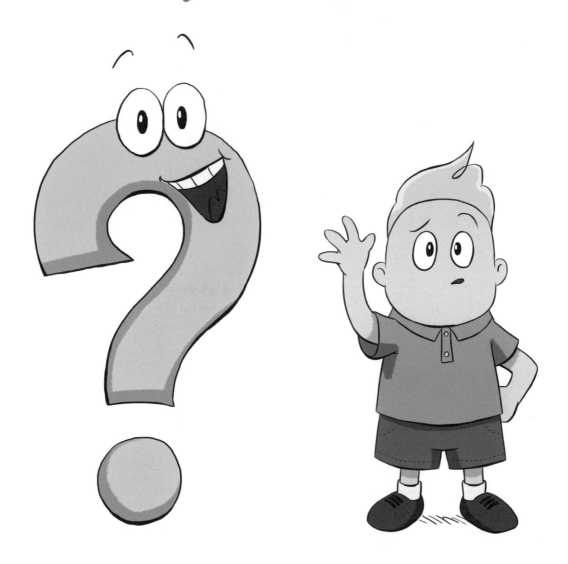

#1. What is the Human Body made of?

a. Jelly Beans
b. Cells
c. Water
d. Bananas

The correct answer is:

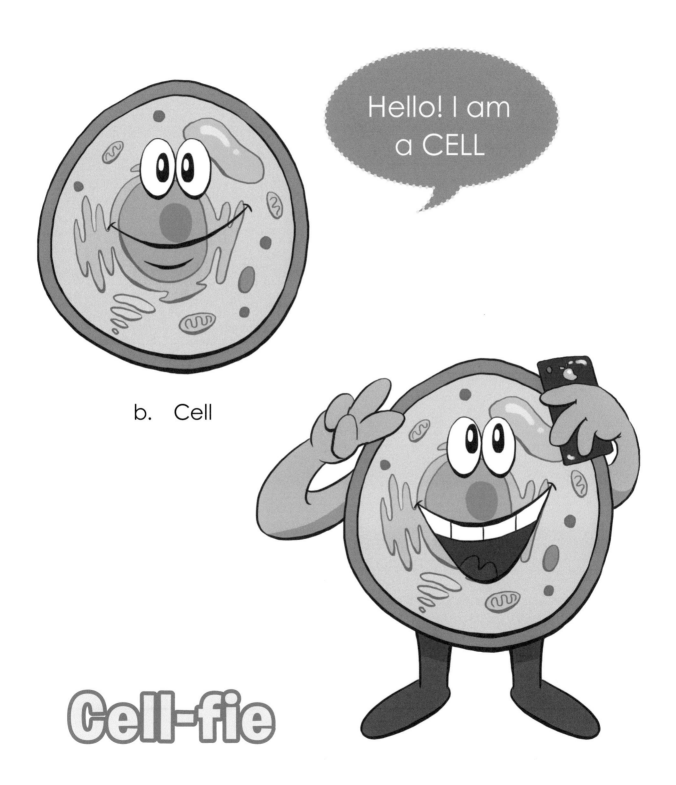

b. Cell

Cell-fie

Question

How many cells do we have in our body?

a.   One Big Cell
b.   Many Hundreds
c.   Many Billions
d.   Many Trillions

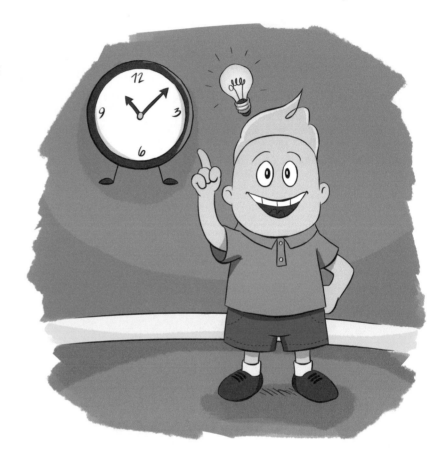

The correct answer is:

d. Many Trillions

One Trillion is 1,000,000 x 1,000,000

1,000,000,000,000

MIND BLOWING FACTS

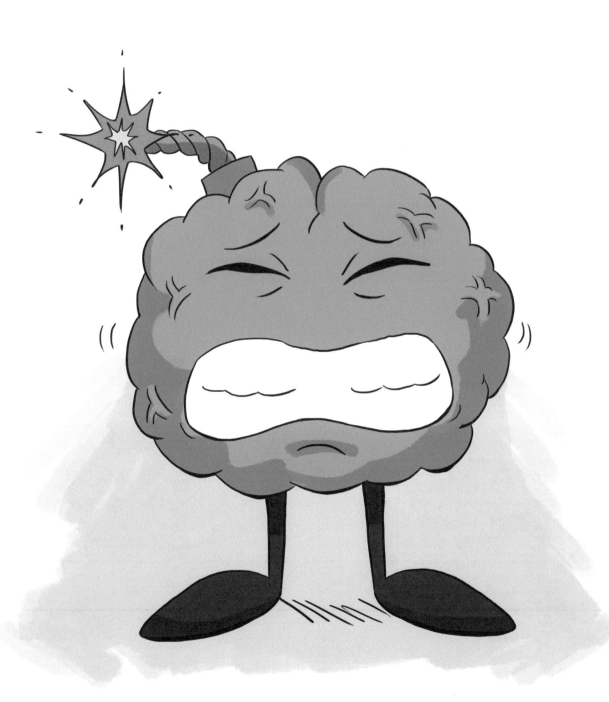

We have many trillions of these living creatures living in us

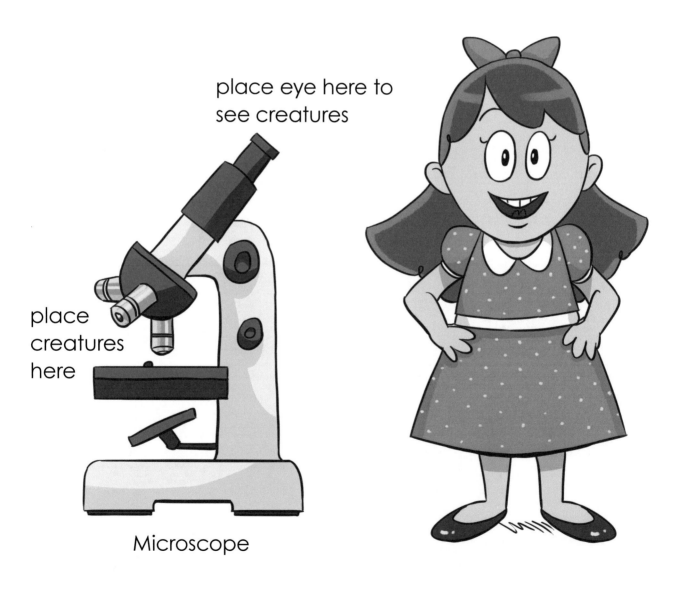

place eye here to see creatures

place creatures here

Microscope

Under the Microscope...

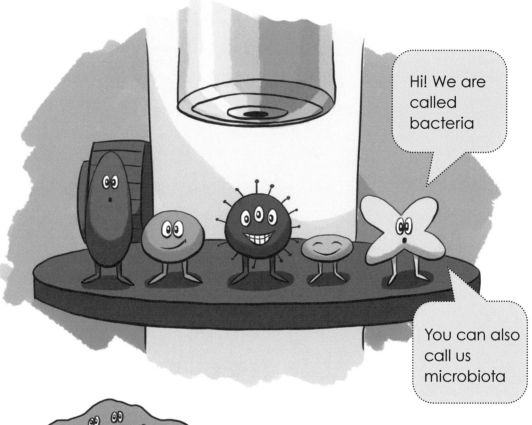

Hi! We are called bacteria

You can also call us microbiota

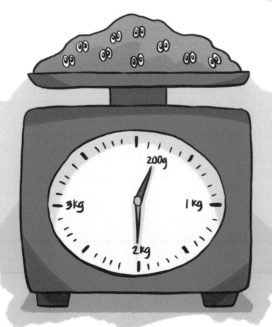

These bacteria can weigh somewhere between 200g to 2 kilograms

Our body is like a house to these microbiota

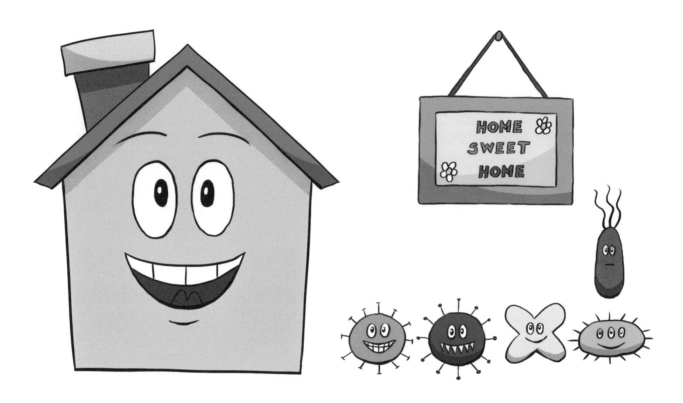

We have many trillions of microbiota in us.

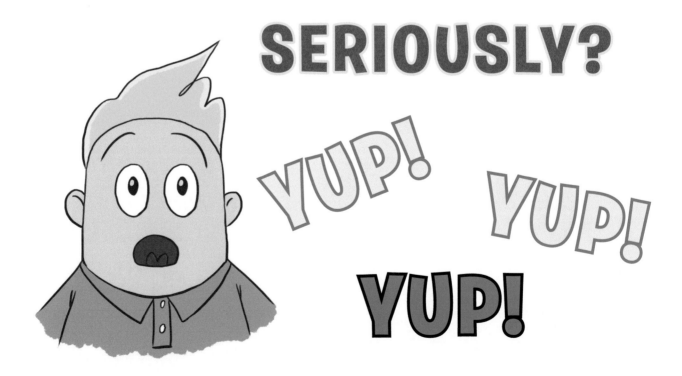

SERIOUSLY?

YUP!

YUP!

YUP!

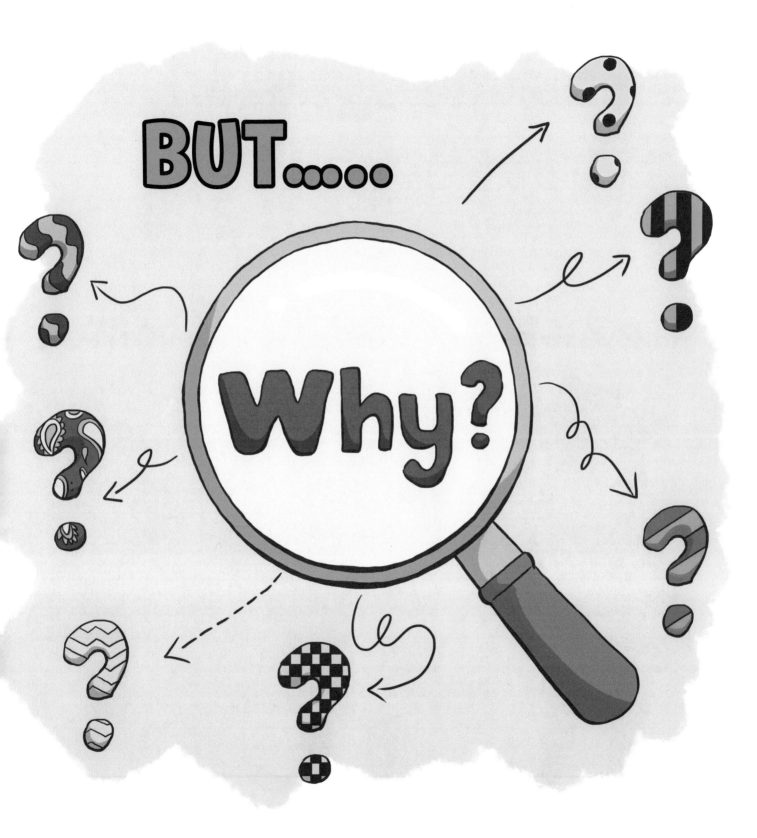

In our world, we have different types of occupations like...

POLICE **CHEF** **DOCTOR**

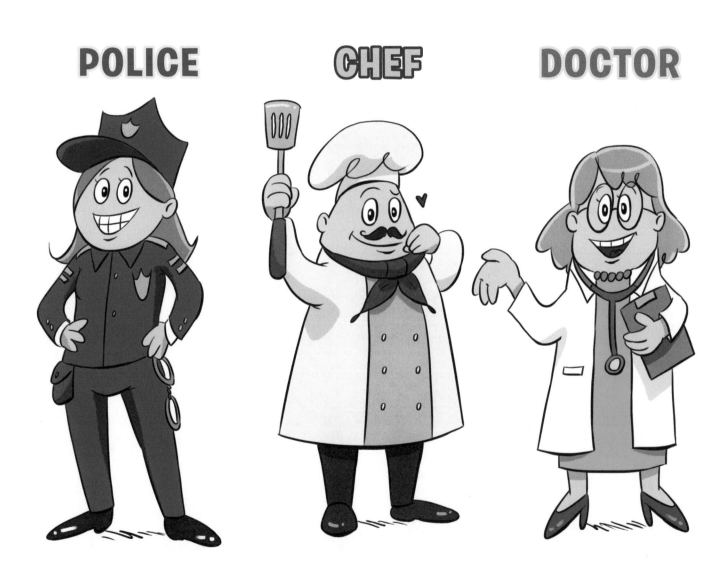

In the microbiota world, different microbiota have different occupations or jobs too. They are super SUPER SUPER important.
Did I mention that our microbiota is

SUPER IMPORTANT???

Here are some of the many many many many many many many many many many many many many many many things or jobs that they do…

IN THE GUT

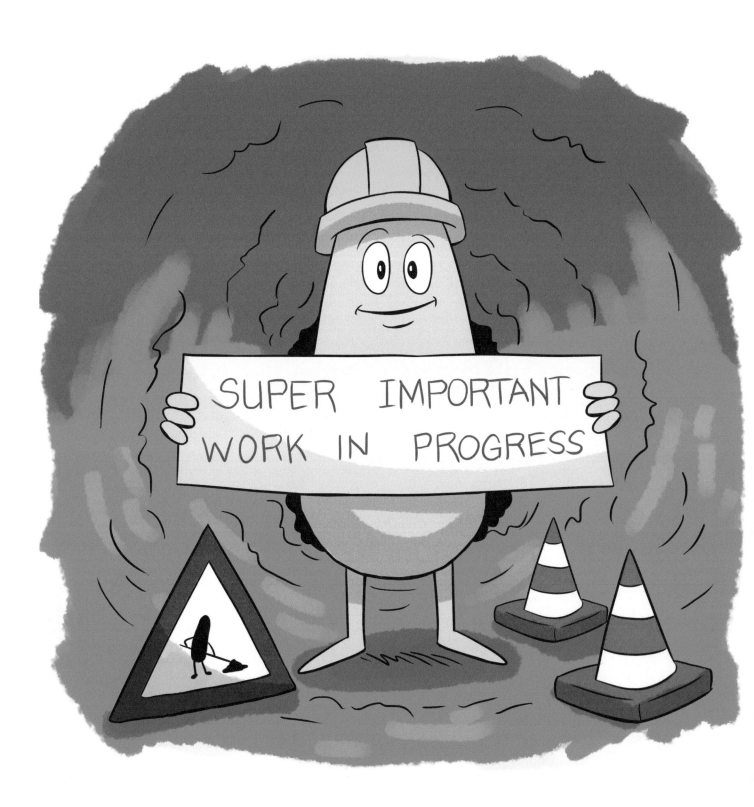

STILL IN THE GUT

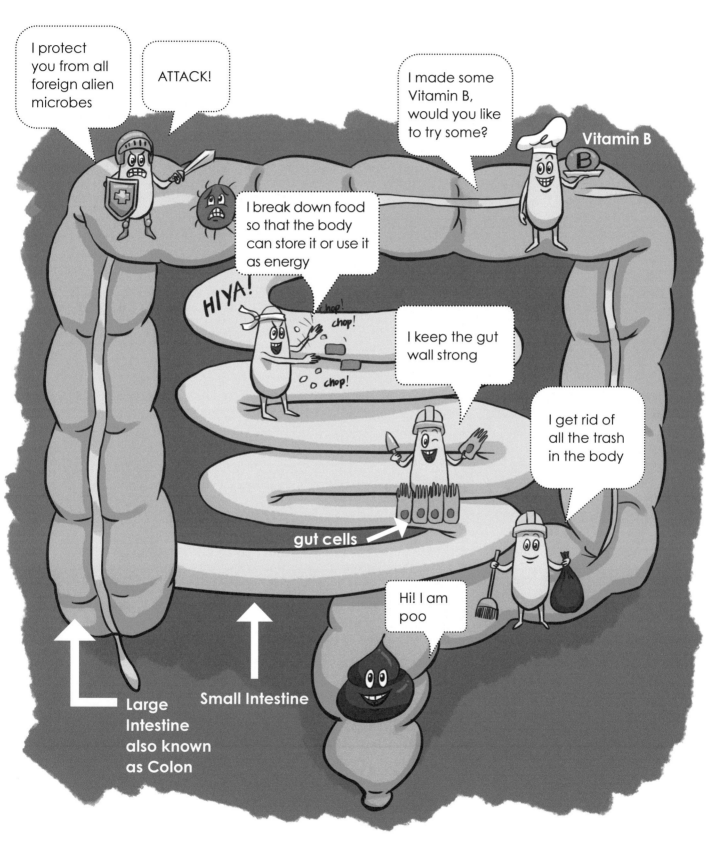

Question

Do your gut microbiota affect how you feel?

a. No
b. Yes
c. Oh look! There's a butterfly

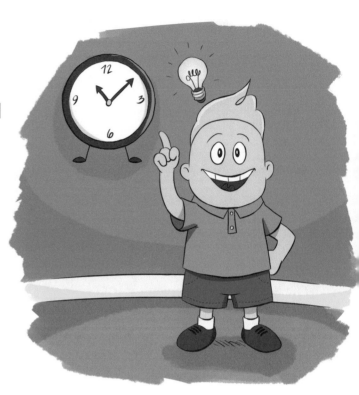

Answer is:

b. Yes

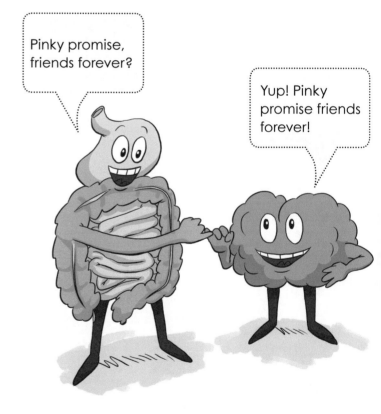

Turns out that the brain and the gut are connected

This is going to sound a little crazy. When we eat good food, we feed good microbes. They grow, multiply and they do their jobs properly.

GOOD FOOD

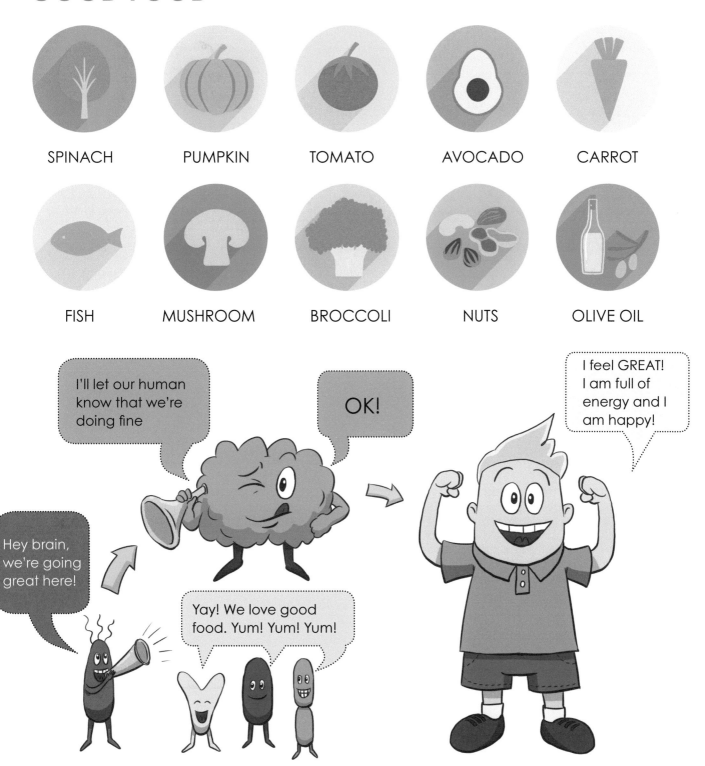

SPINACH   PUMPKIN   TOMATO   AVOCADO   CARROT

FISH   MUSHROOM   BROCCOLI   NUTS   OLIVE OIL

When we eat bad food, we feed the bad microbes. When the bad microbes outnumber the good microbes, we are IN TROUBLE!!!

BAD FOOD

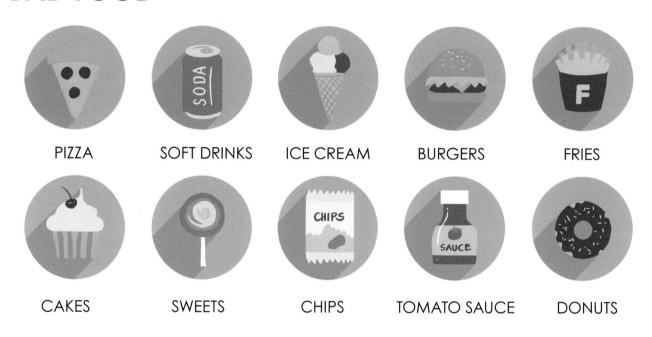

PIZZA   SOFT DRINKS   ICE CREAM   BURGERS   FRIES

CAKES   SWEETS   CHIPS   TOMATO SAUCE   DONUTS

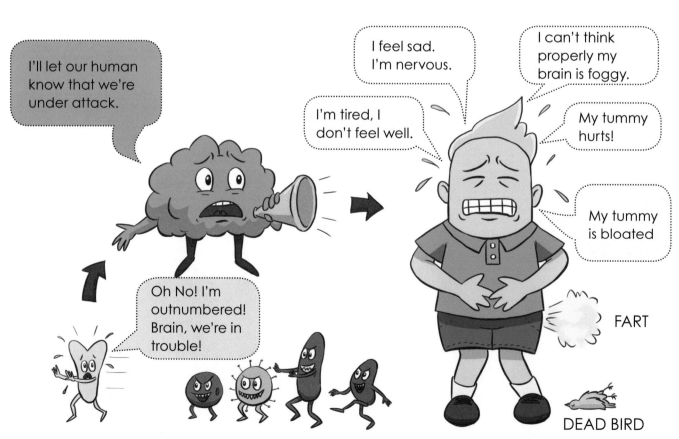

So it's really really really really important to eat healthy food. Good food will feed the right microbiota, they can then do their job properly and keep us healthy. Take care of them and they'll take care of us.

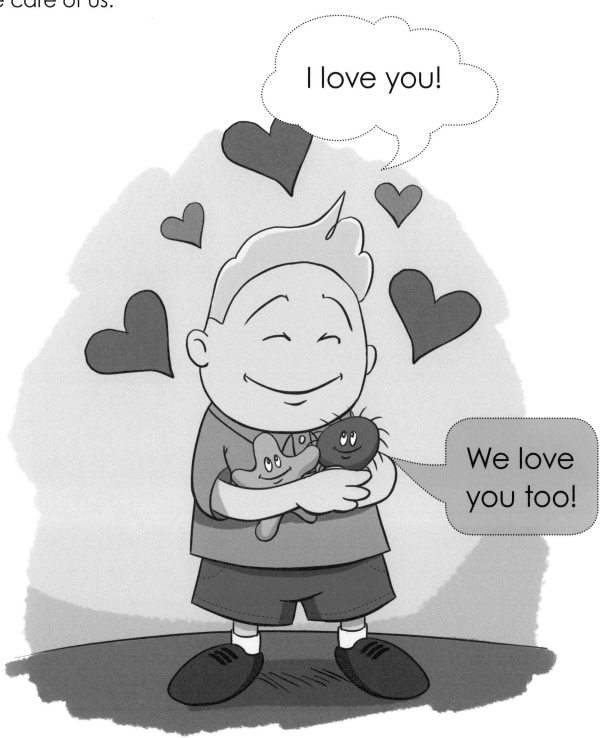

THE END

Printed in the United States
By Bookmasters